Erasing the Ink:
Getting Rid of Your Tattoo

Frank Spalding

ROSEN
PUBLISHING®

New York

Published in 2012 by The Rosen Publishing Group, Inc.
29 East 21st Street, New York, NY 10010

First Edition

Library of Congress Cataloging-in-Publication Data

Spalding, Frank.
Erasing the ink: getting rid of your tattoo / Frank Spalding.—1st ed.
  p. cm.—(Tattooing)
Includes bibliographical references and index.
ISBN 978-1-4488-4615-3 (library binding)
ISBN 978-1-4488-4619-1 (pbk)
ISBN 978-1-4488-4740-2 (6-pack)
1. Skin—Laser surgery. 2. Tattooing. I. Title.
RL120.L37S63 2012
617.4'770598—dc22

2010045920

Manufactured in Malaysia

CPSIA Compliance Information: Batch #S11YA: For further information, contact Rosen Publishing, New York, New York, at 1-800-237-9932.

On the cover: Tattoo removal is a long, painful, and often expensive process. Currently, lasers are the most common method of tattoo removal. These lasers work by breaking the ink into tiny fragments using highly concentrated light.

Contents

INTRODUCTION

People have been getting tattoos for thousands of years. Originally, tattoos had ceremonial purposes or were intended to show an individual's status within his or her community. Today, many cultures and sub-cultures still use tattoos to indicate rank and standing. For instance, it is common for gang members to get tattoos, and Russian prisoners often sport tattoos that indicate their crimes, rank in the underworld, and how much time they have served in prison.

In North America today, most people get tattoos just for fun. For a few hundred dollars, any adult can pay a tattoo artist to ink a design into his or her skin. According to a 2010 Pew Research Center report, 38 percent of U.S. citizens from the ages of seventeen to twenty-nine have tattoos. Tattoos aren't simply for the young, however; the same report revealed that approximately 32 percent of people ages thirty to forty-five are also inked. Since tattoos have gone mainstream, many people get them without giving too much thought as to how much they will like their tattoos several years down the road.

One of the reasons why people get tattoos is that they want permanent markings—the ink won't simply wash off. Getting a tattoo is a commitment, and that in and of itself is a statement. For instance, it is common for people to get the name of a boyfriend or girlfriend tattooed on them. If they stay with that person for the rest of their life, their tattoo is a display of their love and commitment. If they break up, however, the person who had that name tattooed on him or her might not want it anymore. However, tattoos are not meant to be removed. Getting rid of an unwanted tattoo can be time consuming, expensive, and painful. In the world of tattoos, changing one's mind comes at a cost.

Tattoo removal may be difficult, but it isn't impossible. Laser removal is the most common way to remove tattoos. Although laser removal can be somewhat painful, it generally produces the best results. However, laser removal isn't the only option. Intense pulsed light therapy, surgical excision, and dermabrasion are used less often, but they can also be effective. Another option is to get a cover-up tattoo, hiding unwanted ink beneath a new design.

Anyone considering getting a tattoo should think it through very carefully. A tattoo design that seems cool at the moment might not be so appealing in a few years. If that same design had been applied with body paint, henna, or some other temporary tattoo method, rather than being inked directly into the skin with a tattoo gun, it could be removed with little more than soap and water. Getting permanent ink is not a decision to be made on a whim. But if it's too late and that ink needs to be erased, there are options.

Removing Tattoos

Much like a painter creates art on a canvas, a tattoo artist creates art on people's skin. However, if a painter makes a mistake, he or she can easily paint over it—or throw away the canvas altogether. Tattoo artists cannot do this, as their canvas is a living person! Getting rid of a tattoo involves getting the ink out of the person's skin.

So why are tattoos so hard to remove? After all, it's just ink, right? Why should it be so hard to erase? To understand how the process of tattoo removal works and why it is so difficult, we first need to examine how tattoos are placed into the skin.

Under the Skin

The skin is the largest organ of the human body. It performs a number of complicated functions, from regulating body temperature to keeping moisture inside the body. The outer layer of human skin is called the epidermis. The epidermis is thin and waterproof, and it

Laser removal surgery is the most common form of tattoo removal. Lasers penetrate the skin and break up ink trapped in the dermis, fading or erasing the tattoo.

actually contains no blood vessels. The main job of the epidermis is to protect the body from getting an infection. When someone is getting inked, the tattoo artist isn't putting the ink into his or her epidermis. The needle of the tattoo gun penetrates the epidermis and injects the ink directly into the layer of skin below, known as the dermis.

The dermis holds the ink of a tattoo. It is full of a lot of other stuff as well—hair follicles, blood vessels, sweat glands, and more. The needle of a tattoo gun punctures the dermis thousands of times per minute, injecting enough ink into the dermis to create a design that is visible through the epidermis. Trapped inside the skin, a tattoo will last the entirety of a person's life. In fact, some Egyptian mummies have tattoos that are still recognizable after thousands of years!

Tattoo Mistakes

The importance of carefully choosing a tattoo—and its placement—cannot be overstated. Many people get sick of their tattoos simply because they made a foolish tattoo choice, or they got their tattoo on a part of their body, such as the neck or hands, which can't be concealed with clothing. As a result, they may find that they cannot get a job. Still other people pick a tattoo that they think will be perfect, save up their money for it, and couldn't be more excited about walking into the tattoo parlor to get it. But when the tattoo gun stops buzzing and the tattoo artist swabs off the skin a final time and gives them a mirror to take a look at their new

Hidden Dangers

The ink used by professional tattoo parlors is much safer than that used by amateur tattoo artists, who often simply use India ink—or, even worse, break open a ballpoint pen. Still, even the high-quality tattoo ink used by professionals has not been approved by the U.S. Food and Drug Administration (FDA). Some people have allergic reactions to tattoo ink. According to the *New York Times*, some European researchers believe that when tattoo ink is broken up by lasers, it can sometimes create dangerous, possibly carcinogenic, or cancer-causing, by-products that are absorbed by the body. It is a good idea to talk to a doctor about the possible harmful side effects of getting a tattoo—or getting a tattoo removed.

tattoo, these people don't see the design that they wanted. Instead, they see a botched piece of art—much different from the tattoo design they created (or picked off the wall of the shop). Lines that should be straight are wavy, parts of the shading look like giant bleeding wounds, and it just looks horrible overall.

Some tattoo artists are more skilled at their art than others. With tattooing, like any other trade, the more practice an artist gets, the better he or she becomes. In this case, practice involves permanently inking tattoos into people's skin! An inexperienced or careless tattoo artist might screw up the design of a tattoo or place a tattoo too deep. Tattoos placed too deep into the dermis are extremely painful and can look

Some people get custom tattoos. Others simply walk into a tattoo shop and choose a design off the wall. Before getting inked, it's a good idea to make sure that the tattoo artist is skilled and that the tattoo design is not too diffi-cult to execute.

faded after they heal. In addition, the design can be slightly raised on the skin. And even if the tattoo is completely removed, it is very possible that a scar will remain.

Where to Go to Get Inked

To avoid a botched tattoo, it is important to choose a good tattoo shop. The two basic requirements for any tattoo shop worth going to is that it is sanitary and that it employs skilled artists. This might sound obvious, but many people are so

It's important to get a tattoo from an artist who uses sterile equipment and practices proper hygiene, including wearing clean gloves.

focused on getting inked that they don't consider all of the things that could go wrong. Regretting a tattoo is one thing, but getting a botched tattoo is another. No one wants the design that he or she was looking forward to cherishing for the rest of his or her life ruined by a tattoo artist with poor technique.

Today, it is easier than ever to get information on businesses. Web sites such as Yelp.com allow anyone to review a place of business, from restaurants to bike shops to tattoo parlors. Although online reviewers are generally not experts in their field, reading a lot of reviews can give someone who desires a tattoo a general idea of what he or she can expect when choosing a tattoo shop.

After locating a shop that looks promising, make sure to visit beforehand and get an idea of the cleanliness of the shop.

Because tattoo artists ink permanent designs into human skin, they must constantly practice in order to improve. This artist is sketching new tattoo designs.

A dirty shop (or a shop with unhygienic tattoo artists) is definitely not a good place to get a tattoo. When a tattoo is first applied, it is essentially a wound on the body, and it should be treated as such. No one would consent to being operated on by a grubby surgeon in a filthy, smoky hospital. And no one should consent to getting a tattoo in a shop that isn't a sterile environment. If the tattoo area becomes infected, it can result in faded-looking ink, scarring, and other complications.

When planning a design, be sure to pick something that can be executed properly. Perfectly round circles are difficult for tattoo artists to pull off. In fact, for Japanese calligraphers, the ability to draw a perfect circle marks them as masters of their craft, and calligraphic masters are few and far between. Perfect parallel lines and grids are also extremely difficult for tattoo artists to execute properly.

Finally, it is important to review the tattoo artist's portfolio. A portfolio is a collection of photographs documenting a tattoo artist's work. Tattoo shops should have each artist's portfolio available for customers to look at. If his or her work looks less than stellar, it is best to find a more competent tattoo artist.

A tattoo artist first applies the tattoo design to a customer's skin with a stencil. Then the artist should show the design to the customer before applying it to his or her skin. This is the customer's last chance to look over the design and make sure that he or she still likes it. It is also the customer's last chance to catch any mistakes or spelling errors—nothing is more embarrassing than a misspelled tattoo!

Deciding on Tattoo Removal

There is no sure way to know how one will feel about a tattoo a few years after getting it. A design that seemed like it would make an awesome tattoo sometimes just doesn't look very good when it is inked into one's skin. Also, people's tastes change over time. The stuff that seemed cool when they were younger might not seem so cool as they get older. Just think about it: most seventeen-year-olds like music that is different from what they listened to when they were twelve. They also dress differently, do different things for fun, and have different posters on their walls; tastes can change a lot in five years. The same holds true for tattoos. Though not impossible, the chances are pretty slim that someone will, at the age of twenty-two, still be into a tattoo that he or she got at seventeen. Getting a tattoo is a big deal, and getting a tattoo removed is also a big decision. It is expensive, painful, and inconvenient.

It is difficult to say how long the removal will take. Complicated tattoos with many colors might require more than a dozen visits to remove, and even then it might be impossible to remove them completely. A simple black ink tattoo might require only a couple of visits, but the removal process might leave a visible scar.

Anyone getting a tattoo removed needs to have realistic expectations going into the process. When deciding on tattoo removal, it can be a good idea to talk to someone who has actually gotten a tattoo removed. Find out what the person's experience of tattoo removal was, if he or she has any advice, and if he or she can recommend a good doctor to perform the removal. It can also be helpful to look online for information about tattoo removal. Remember that it can be difficult to verify information found on the Internet, and decisions shouldn't be based solely on online reviews, especially not for something as serious as tattoo removal. Before deciding on anything, it is of paramount importance that anyone wanting to erase ink talk to a doctor.

Some dermatologists and cosmetic surgeons are skilled at tattoo removal. After finding a doctor to perform the procedure, it is important to schedule a consultation to discuss the options. The doctor can estimate how long the removal process will take and explain what to expect when undergoing treatment. Be aware that current tattoo removal technology cannot provide a pain-free tattoo removal experience. This might be possible someday, but it is not possible right now. Any doctor worth visiting should explain what the removal process actually entails, including the unpleasant parts. Anything less would be dishonest.

Laser It Off

Most doctors will recommend laser tattoo removal to people who want to erase their ink. Besides being the most effective and popular form of tattoo removal, laser removal is also the least invasive. It is performed without puncturing the skin.

Lasers

Today, lasers are used in appliances to read information from CDs and DVDs, by police officers to measure how fast cars are going, and by doctors to perform surgery. Some lasers are more specialized than others. For instance, a laser used in a simple laser pointer is very low-intensity, as its function is merely to project a dot onto a nearby surface. A laser used for optical surgery, on the other hand, is designed for precision use.

The lasers used for tattoo removal work by breaking up the tattoo ink stored in the dermis. After the ink molecules are broken up, they are reabsorbed by the body. This causes the tattoo to fade—in some cases, it eventually can be removed completely. A skilled doctor can make sure that the laser targets only areas of the skin where the tattoo ink is stored.

The ability for lasers to be wielded in a controlled manner makes laser tattoo removal a process with many benefits and few drawbacks. It is generally effective, non-invasive, and safe. There is no bleeding, and with the proper care, there is almost no risk of complications following the procedure. Best of all, out of all the varieties of tattoo removal currently available, laser removal leaves the least amount of scarring afterward.

Getting Laser Tattoo Removal

Just as it is important to find a good tattoo artist when getting a tattoo, it is important to shop around and find a good place to remove it. An unlikely source of information might be a local tattoo parlor—few people know more about tattooing than the tattoo artists themselves. They may be able to recommend a trustworthy place to get a tattoo removed. In fact, some tattoo artists may have had tattoos removed themselves! Actual referrals from others who have gotten tattoos removed might be the best way to find a place.

Laser treatment

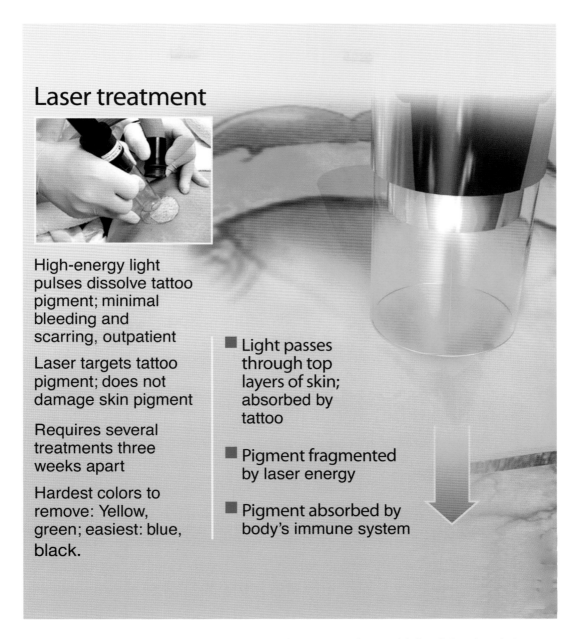

High-energy light pulses dissolve tattoo pigment; minimal bleeding and scarring, outpatient

Laser targets tattoo pigment; does not damage skin pigment

Requires several treatments three weeks apart

Hardest colors to remove: Yellow, green; easiest: blue, black.

- Light passes through top layers of skin; absorbed by tattoo

- Pigment fragmented by laser energy

- Pigment absorbed by body's immune system

Laser treatment can be expensive and may require multiple visits, but it is also the least invasive method of tattoo removal.

Finding a place that performs laser tattoo removal is only the first step, however. Once a likely place has been located, it's good to talk to the person who will be doing the procedure. Ask the person lots of questions, and be sure to find out how experienced he or she is. If he or she is new on the job, it might be better to go somewhere else. Doctors should be willing to answer any questions they are asked, both about the procedure and the equipment they use. As time goes on, tattoo removal technology only grows more and more sophisticated. Ask what kind of equipment is used in the office and research it online—is it currently the most advanced on the market? Or is it obsolete? It's best to go to a place that has the most cutting-edge equipment available.

How Much Is This Going to Cost?

The cost of tattoo removal depends on a number of factors. The first factor in determining the cost is the doctor—everyone has different prices for tattoo removal. Sometimes, this is based on the quality of care. It's possible that a veteran doctor using the most up-to-date equipment might be more expensive than a less experienced doctor. It is very important to talk frankly with the doctor about the cost of the removal. Tattoo removal is generally considered to be elective surgery, which is seldom covered by health insurance. If money is an issue, shop around.

Surgical Lasers

The precise nature of lasers makes them ideal for surgical use. Today, surgeons around the world use lasers. Surgical lasers can cut and cauterize flesh, as well as penetrate the skin without making an incision. Surgeries that used to be extremely invasive and require a great deal of recovery time have been greatly simplified, thanks to lasers. For instance, the surgical removal of cataracts from the eye used to be very painful and required that the patient keep his or her eyes bandaged for days. Today, cataract removal is generally an outpatient surgery, meaning the patient gets to go home the same day. It is expected that laser technology will continue to advance, becoming even more sophisticated than it is now.

The most significant factor in calculating the cost of removing a tattoo is the size and complexity of the tattoo. Large tattoos simply take longer to remove, which equals more work for the person performing the procedure. In addition, not all tattoo inks can be effectively removed by the same kind of laser. Doctors may have to use different lasers on different kinds of inks. Different colors of ink respond to different wavelengths of laser, so the removal of multicolored tattoos can be fairly complicated.

Generally, amateur tattoos are easier to remove than professional ones. Some amateur artists use tattoo guns, but most simply wrap a needle in some thread, dip it in ink, and apply the tattoo by stabbing the skin over and over again! This usually results in a pretty lousy tattoo. It also means that the ink is not all set in the dermis at the same depth and is less uniform, making it less difficult for doctors to target the ink with a laser.

Another factor in determining the cost of tattoo removal is how many visits it will take. Large or complex tattoos will probably require multiple visits. It is likely that the price quoted will be per treatment, as opposed to a flat rate for the full removal of the tattoo. Sometimes, it's possible for a doctor to be able to estimate how many treatments will be needed to laser off a tattoo. More often, though, a doctor will need to see how the tattoo responds to

Tattoos with multiple colors can look great—but they are more complicated to remove. The different colors each might require a different type of laser.

treatment. Still, some tattoos can be more stubborn than others. Even the kind of tattoo ink used can influence the removal process.

Despite these variables, a doctor should be able to set a price for each treatment and hopefully be able to estimate how many treatments the entire process will take. Yet there is no telling how many treatments will go into any given removal process. Tattoo removal can run into the thousands of dollars.

Tattoo removal can also be time consuming. Multiple visits are usually necessary, and typically, it's recommended that each visit is a month apart. It might take more than a year to fully remove the tattoo. Each treatment usually takes only a few minutes, although treating a large tattoo might take thirty to forty-five minutes. Many doctors will inject the area of the removal site with the painkiller lidocaine. Patients have the right to request anesthetics such as lidocaine if they want a relatively pain-free procedure. During the procedure, patients lie on a table or sit in a chair, and wear dark glasses to protect their eyes from harmful light.

Q-switched Lasers

Most clinics use Q-switched lasers to remove tattoos. These types of lasers produce intense pulses of energy for very brief periods of time, sometimes for only nanoseconds. Different kinds of Q-switched lasers are effective on different kinds of tattoo pigments. (They can also be used to target other skin pigments, such as age spots.)

Q-switched ruby lasers and Q-switched alexandrite lasers are often used on darker tattoo pigments, such as black, blue, and green inks. These lasers can also remove melanin, or naturally occurring skin pigments. To lessen this effect, some physicians use Q-switched Nd:YAG lasers (the name of this laser is an acronym for "neodymium-doped yttrium aluminum garnet"). These lasers tend to be effective on red, orange, and yellow inks as well. Black ink absorbs nearly all kinds of light, so it is the easiest color to remove. Colors such as yellow and green, however, can be trickier to remove. Lasers that are gentler on the skin's natural pigment may leave less of a mark but require more treatments in order to remove the tattoo.

Some of the newest tattoo removal technologies allow doctors to switch between different kinds of lasers with a single machine, called the VersaPulse C. The VersaPulse C is generally effective in removing different colors of tattoo ink, and it has a cooling system that minimizes damage to the epidermis, resulting in less skin damage from the treatment.

Aftercare

After each session, it is important to take proper care of the affected skin. Immediately following treatment, the skin may be red, swollen, and sore. Some people experience bruising. (A cold compress, such as an ice pack, can relieve some of

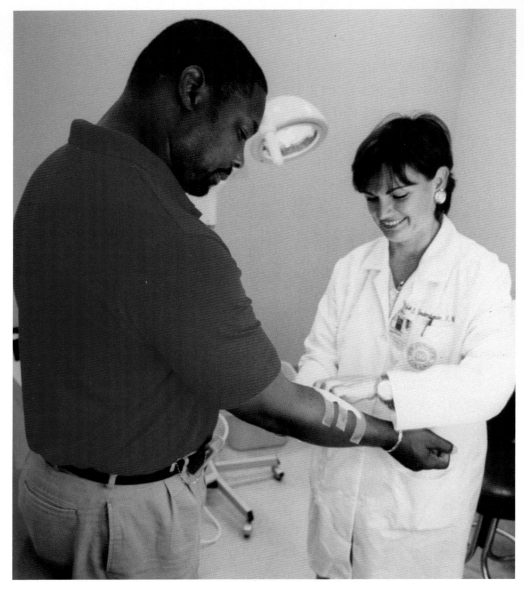

The organization Operation Fresh Start provides gang members with free tattoo removal treatments to remove their gang tattoos. Seen here is Roland Harper, who once played pro football for the Chicago Bears and now assists the program.

this discomfort.) It's not uncommon to discover that scabs or blisters have formed over the affected area. Also, the area that has been treated might appear to be lightened. Usually, this is only temporary.

Much like it's best to treat new tattoos like injuries until they are properly healed, it's important to take good care of tattoos undergoing the process of laser removal. This can help prevent infection and lessen the chance of complications. Talk to a physician to see what kinds of bandages, dressings, and medications should be purchased in order to care for the affected area. Doctors will often recommend topical antibiotics as well as gauze and medical tape to cover the tattoo.

Depending on the size and location of the tattoo being removed, there is a chance that certain activities will need to be avoided until the healing process is complete. Many of the activities that should be avoided are the same as those that would be foregone after first getting a tattoo: so no swimming for a while, avoiding direct sunlight, no aspirin (which can worsen bleeding or bruising), and no applying of any medications to the affected area that are not first recommended or approved by your physician. Also, avoid irritating the affected area by picking at it or scratching it. Although the area will probably heal in about six to eight weeks, it's a good idea to cover it for three months with sunblock that has an SPF rating of no less than 25. This can help prevent the affected area from getting sun damaged, while allowing the skin to breathe, free of a bandage.

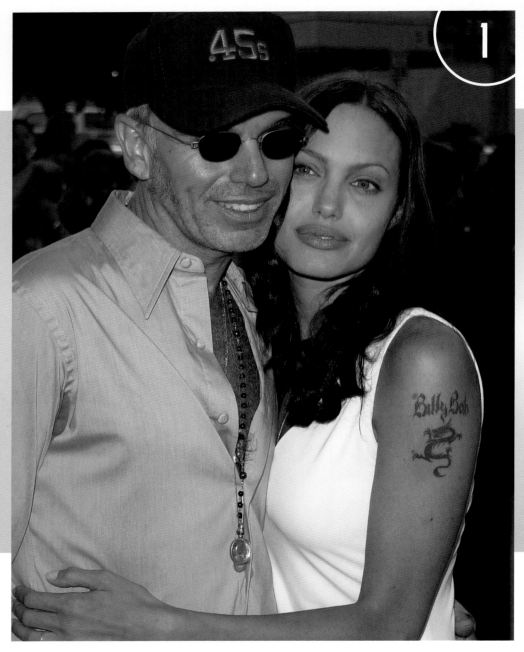

1

Actress Angelina Jolie is seen here in 2001 alongside her then husband Billy Bob Thornton, whose first name she had tattooed on her arm.

2

Jolie and Thornton's marriage did not last. After they divorced, Jolie had his name removed from her tattoo, as seen here.

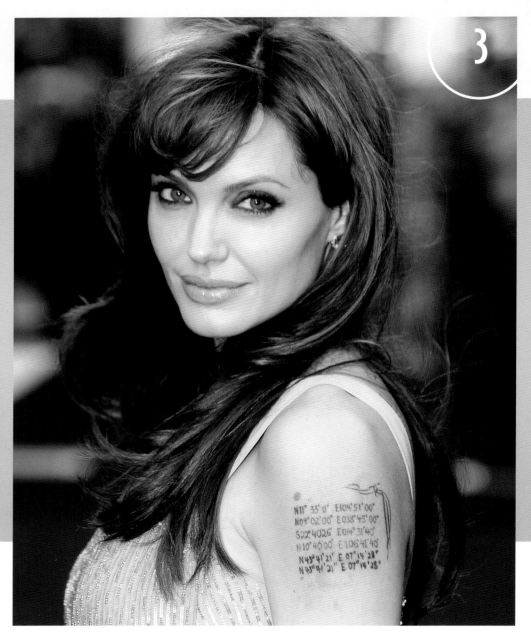

3

By 2010, Jolie had decided to remove her entire old tattoo and get a new one. The new tattoo lists the latitudes and longitudes of the birthplaces of her children. The old dragon tattoo is still barely visible beneath the new tattoo.

Side Effects

Because laser removal is totally noninvasive, many people optimistically hope that their skin will look exactly the way that it did before they got the tattoo. Sadly, this is seldom the case. While it is often possible to completely remove tattoos, it is rare that they can be removed without leaving some sort of mark. After the post-removal scabs and blisters heal completely, it's possible to take a look at how the skin will appear in the long run. Sometimes, laser removal procedures cause scarring or they permanently lighten the skin. Other times, the procedures can actually change the texture of the skin. Of course, everyone who wants his or her tattoos removed hopes for the best—that the skin will look exactly the way it did…almost as if he or she had never gotten a tattoo. Remember, the decision to get a tattoo should not be taken lightly. Once that tattoo is inked, your skin will never be the same again.

Some people choose to use laser removal to progressively lighten their tattoos until they can be covered up with other tattoos. Others find that their tattoos simply do not respond to laser removal, so they need to opt for a different kind of procedure, which can include dermabrasion and excision. Others decide to try their luck with newer treatment procedures, such as intense pulsed light therapy.

Other Tattoo Removal Methods

New technologies promise to revolutionize the field of tattoo removal. New laser technologies could make lasers more precise. Some companies are working on creating creams that could be applied to the surface of the skin to remove the tattoo. Many hope that the day will come when technology will permit tattoos to be removed completely, with little pain or other negative side effects. Right now, however, there are only a few proven tattoo removal methods besides laser removal. These are intense pulsed light therapy, excision, and dermabrasion.

Intense Pulsed Light Therapy

Intense pulsed light (IPL) therapy is used by dermatologists to remove skin blemishes, such as age spots and moles. Although sometimes confused with laser removal, IPL therapy is somewhat different. Instead of a laser, this form of therapy uses intense light to penetrate the skin. And unlike laser removal, a gel is

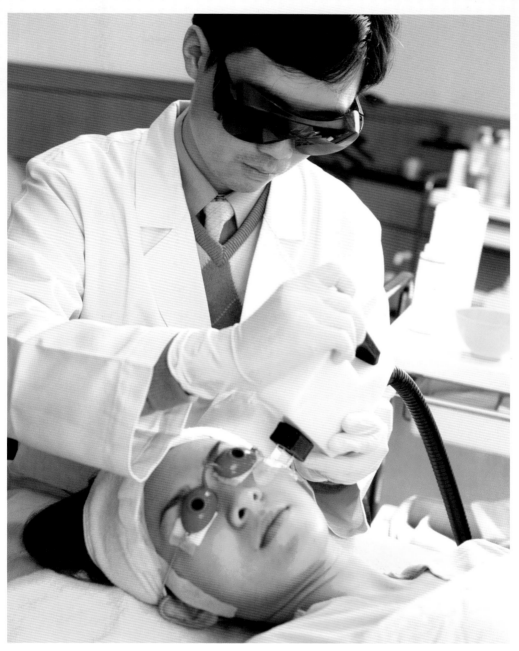

This woman is undergoing a surgical treatment performed with the use of lasers. She has to wear special goggles to protect her eyes from harm.

applied over the area to be treated before it is hit with pulses of light. Proponents of IPL therapy believe that the pulses of light can be adjusted more precisely for individual patients.

Like laser removal, however, IPL therapy is painful. Some patients opt for anesthesia to lessen the pain of the light pulses. Some say that IPL therapy is more effective than laser removal, but it isn't ideal for all patients. In some cases, it can cause an uneven increase in skin pigmentation, and patients with darker skin tones usually experience complications. Usually, candidates for IPL treatment first undergo a test treatment, where a single pulse of light is applied to a patch of skin to see if there will be any unwanted pigmentation side effects. Also, people who take blood-thinning medication or who are diabetics cannot receive IPL treatment.

Tattoo Removal Programs

For former gang members, tattoo removal can be serious business. Many of them get gang-related tattoos—often done by amateurs—when they are in their teens. Sometimes, this is part of the gang initiation. For those who want to move on and put their time as a gang member behind them, these tattoos can be a major obstacle to establishing life in the legitimate world. Employers already can be hesitant to hire people with visible tattoos, never mind visible tattoos that indicate an allegiance to a gang. Furthermore, having these tattoos can make them a target for rival gang members.

Tattoo removal is expensive—often much too expensive for young people to be able to afford. To help offset the costs, some organizations have created programs to pay for the removal of gang tattoos. Sometimes, the cost of removing the tattoo is provided outright; other times, applicants for this program are required to undergo counseling or perform community service in return for the removal treatments or a discount on tattoo removal fees. These programs generally favor laser tattoo removal.

Operation Fresh Start founder Dr. Jay Rosenberg removes a Latin Queen gang tattoo. For former gang members, getting a gang tattoo removed can be an important part of building a new life.

It is believed that IPL treatments can remove tattoos in fewer sessions than laser treatments can. Good news, right? However, there is a major drawback to IPL therapy, even for those who are eligible for it: the price. Most places charge for each pulse of light, rather than per session. This means that the size of the tattoo being removed is a major factor in how much its removal will cost. The cost of each pulse can run upward of $10. Also, many places have a minimum charge for each visit, which can be more than $100. The fact that IPL therapy is so expensive and not appropriate for all skin types has ensured that laser treatment is still the most commonly used method of tattoo removal. Some people think that IPL therapy may some-day become more popular than laser removal for getting rid of unwanted ink. Should this happen, it's likely that the cost of IPL treatments will drop. Until then, however, it remains one of the most expensive, albeit effective, means of tattoo removal.

Perhaps someday, IPL therapy will be fine-tuned to the extent that everyone can benefit from it. In the meantime, it is definitely an option for people with very fair skin. It is rare that IPL therapy results in scabs or bleeding, although sometimes the skin of the affected area undergoes pigmentation changes, becoming lighter or darker.

Excision

Prior to the invention of noninvasive forms of tattoo removal, there was no "easy" way to get rid of a tattoo. Since doctors could not target the tattoo ink in the skin, their only recourse was to simply remove the skin where the tattoo was. Although rarely used today, surgical excision can be effective in removing tattoos that won't respond to any other form of treatment.

Unlike laser removal and IPL therapy, excision is extremely invasive and must be performed by a surgeon. The doctor performing the surgery uses a scalpel to cut the tattoo out of the patient's skin and then closes the wound. Sometimes, an inflatable sac is inserted under the skin and blown up, stretching the skin of the tattoo in order to allow surgeons to remove it with greater precision. Because of how invasive this procedure is, few people opt for it as their first choice. Excision always leaves a scar, although some people are more prone to scarring than others. The scar left by excision depends largely on the size of the tattoo and its location on the body.

Excision works better on small tattoos than on large ones. Because it is cheaper than laser removal, some people with smaller tattoos simply elect to get them excised. Sure, it may leave a scar, but it takes only a single visit and it's easier on the wallet. However, like other forms of tattoo removal, excision is considered elective surgery and, therefore, is not covered by most forms of health insurance. As such, it is important to have a frank talk with the doctor about the costs of the procedure and to make sure that he or she can competently perform the procedure.

Dermabrasion

Another extremely invasive tattoo removal procedure is known as dermabrasion. This procedure involves the use of a spinning disk that basically grinds layers of skin away. Generally, dermabrasion is not the first procedure recommended for tattoo removal. Unlike excision, dermabrasion usually requires several sessions to yield results. And while it takes only seven to ten days for the scabbed-over skin to heal, it will remain visibly red or pink for two to three months. Beyond that, it can take up to six months to truly be able to gauge the final result of the treatments. This treatment was not originally designed with tattoo removal in mind. Instead, it was to help correct skin damaged by acne scars or other blemishes, as the skin generally grows back smoother after this procedure.

It is unlikely that a doctor would recommend dermabrasion to remove a tattoo, but it is possible. Some see dermabrasion as a sort of compromise between laser removal and excision. It's definitely important to go to an experienced surgeon, ask a lot of questions, and ensure that the doctor takes a thorough medical history.

For many people, the initially cosmetically hideous results of dermabrasion are a major downside of the procedure. However, after the scab has healed, there are steps that can be taken to make the skin appear more even-toned until the healing process is complete. For instance, some people use hypoallergenic makeup to even out the skin tone in the affected area. During the healing process, it is important to keep the affected area out of the sun or cover it with a sun-block that has an SPF of at least 25.

Saline Injections

Saline injections can help lighten existing tattoos. Saline is a completely sterile solution of sodium chloride in water. In a very simple procedure, the saline is injected into an existing tattoo. Sometimes, this can work to break up the tattoo, effectively making it fade. The benefits of getting saline injections are that they involve almost no risk if performed properly, are much less painful than other methods, and are minimally invasive. In addition, the recovery time is more or less equal to the recovery time of getting a tattoo.

Getting saline injections is generally cheaper than other tattoo removal methods. However, this procedure cannot fully remove a tattoo. Instead, it can effectively "blur" the old tattoo, making it easier for a cover-up tattoo to be applied. There is little chance that saline injections will result in changes of the skin's texture and pigmentation or result in any scarring. The results can be a bit unpredictable, but many people who opt for saline injections are of the opinion that there is little to lose by trying them out.

Proceed with Caution: Unproven Removal Methods

It is absolutely necessary to consult with qualified, experienced dermatologists and other doctors before choosing a method of tattoo removal. Tattoo removal is always expensive and is frequently painful. There is no getting around these facts. Searching for qualified doctors with the latest equipment can take time and patience, and getting the proper treatment costs money—and these costs will most likely not be reimbursed by health insurance. Some removal methods produce unsightly scabs and blisters, which makes some people uneasy. Simply put, getting a tattoo removed is a massive inconvenience, and many people are tempted to seek out alternative treatments that are easier and less expensive than proven tattoo removal methods.

There are a number of products out there—many of which are being sold only on the Internet—that claim to remove tattoos cheaply, quickly, and painlessly. The overwhelming

Sometimes, doctors inject saline solution under the skin to lighten a tattoo before beginning laser removal treatments.

majority of these products have not undergone proper tests and have not been approved by the FDA. They may be hazardous to one's health, and little evidence exists to prove that they actually work. After all, if they worked the way they promised, surely they would be just as popular as laser removal.

Some of the most common products that promise to erase unwanted ink are tattoo removal creams. Most of these products claim that they can fade tattoos by simply being applied topically on the skin. Unless a doctor recommends these creams, they should be regarded with suspicion at the very least and should probably be avoided altogether.

Living with the Results

The tattoo removal process can be long and arduous. It is easy to be self-conscious about the faded, scabbed-over tattoo that is in the process of being lasered off. The removal process can also be strange. Most people getting a tattoo removed are doing so for the first time and, therefore, may be wary about undergoing a medical procedure. Post-procedure, they may worry that the side effects of their treatment are abnormal.

For these reasons, it can be a good idea to reach out to others who have gone through the same process. Talking to friends or acquaintances who have gotten tattoos removed is a good step, as is joining online tattoo removal support groups. If participating in an online group, remember that maintaining one's privacy online is important above all else. It's never a good idea to share personal information or photographs with strangers on the Internet.

Tattoo removal isn't always pretty. Here, a laser removal treatment has resulted in a giant wound, which may leave a nasty scar.

Coping with Scars

Everyone who goes to get a tattoo removed hopes for the best. Sometimes, however, tattoo removal can result in scars and other skin blemishes. For many people, a scar is preferable to an unwanted tattoo. Scars from tattoo removal can be divided into two categories: hypertrophic scars and keloids.

Hypertrophic scars occur when skin that is regenerating grows larger cells than normal. As a result, the scars appear to be slightly raised. In time, hypertrophic scars can fade away and even be tattooed over. Keloid scars, however, are more severe. They are noticeably raised from the surrounding skin and are firm to the touch. They can even get worse if they are subjected to further injury, which means that they cannot be tattooed over. Generally, people with dark skin are more prone to developing keloid scars as a result of tattoo removal surgery than people with fair skin. The more severe an injury, the greater the chance that scars will form as a result. The formation of scars is influenced by a number of factors, including the severity of the wound, the individual's age, and the location of the scar on his or her body.

Many people with scars want to remove them—or at least reduce the appearance of them. Unfortunately, there is only so much that can be done to accomplish this, and anyone hoping to fade or otherwise reduce the scarring should be realistic about what the results will be. Scars can be made smaller surgically, although this is often carried out only in extreme cases. Sometimes, they can be reduced with treatments such as laser therapy and dermabrasion, as well as steroid injections. As a simple measure, protecting scars with sunscreen can help make them less visible, as scars don't tan the way the surrounding skin does.

Many over-the-counter creams and ointments claim to fade scars, but the FDA hasn't reviewed a good number of them. People who are looking for products that will effectively reduce the appearance of scars should use only those that are recommended by their physician.

Getting a Cover-up Tattoo

Tattoo artists can often cover up unwanted or inexpertly applied tattoos with new tattoos. For people who don't mind having a tattoo but want to get rid of the one they have, cover-ups can be a good option. Some tattoo artists excel at doing cover-up tattoos, and their work can be extremely effective. If everything goes well, the unwanted tattoo can be completely covered with a new design. Skilled artists can also "correct" poorly done tattoos.

Anyone thinking of getting a cover-up tattoo should research prospective tattoo artists very carefully. It's best to go to an artist who has a reputation for doing effective cover-up jobs. Make sure that the artist's reputation is backed up by a solid portfolio of before-and-after photographs of his or her work. It is important to talk with the artist about cover-up options and make sure that one is completely happy with the design before getting the work done. After all, no one wants a bad cover-up tattoo! Imagine how annoying it would be to get a tattoo to cover a tattoo that's covering a tattoo. Unfortunately, this may leave an enormous amount of pigment in one site that a laser cannot ever remove effectively.

Cover-up tattoos will always be larger than the designs they cover—usually significantly so. They also tend to use a lot of dark colors and black shading, which will help obscure the old, unwanted design. In addition, most cover-up tattoos need to be custom-designed in order to fit the needs of the

Using concealer can be an easy, inexpensive, and convenient way to temporarily cover up a tattoo. It's important for those buying concealer to make sure that it matches their skin tone.

job. The tattoo being covered presents the tattoo artist with certain limitations as to what the new design can be.

Sometimes, a tattoo artist will recommend undergoing a session or two of laser removal treatments to fade the tattoo being covered up. This is especially true for tattoos that are large or have a lot of dark ink. Some tattoos, however, may not be able to be effectively covered.

Simple Tattoo Cover-up Methods

The most inexpensive way to erase a tattoo is to simply cover it with clothing or makeup. Tattoos that are not on the face or hands can usually be hidden pretty easily. Some people like their tattoos but may not want to display them in certain types of social situations. For example, they might be afraid that a visible tattoo would be a liability during a job interview. Or, they might not want their great-grandmother to see the tattoo on their forearm. There is nothing inherently wrong with having a tattoo, and there's nothing wrong with wanting to cover up a tattoo on occasion.

Many people use makeup to cover up their tattoos when needed. This can be a somewhat time-consuming process, especially if one is not used to applying makeup. Concealer is a kind of makeup designed to be relatively opaque. It is used to cover blemishes and dark patches of skin. For instance, some people use concealer to cover dark circles under their eyes. Generally, concealer can be applied directly to the skin or over a layer of foundation makeup.

There are actually brands of makeup specifically designed to conceal tattoos, such as Ben Nye Tattoo Cover concealer makeup. Ben Nye is a company that specializes in makeup used by actors in theater or film. Its Tattoo Cover makeup was designed to obscure tattoos. Another brand of makeup is Sephora's Kat Von D Tattoo Concealer, named after the famous tattoo artist. While these brands are marketed specifically for people who want to conceal their ink, it's also possible to simply use regular concealer.

Covering up a tattoo with makeup takes some skill and practice to do well. The first step is finding a concealer that matches one's skin tone. This can be tricky, so it is best done in person at a makeup store. Don't be afraid to talk to store clerks about what shade of concealer would work the best. Ask if there are any samples available for customers to try. Covering dark tattoos can be tricky. Sometimes, the type of concealer that matches a person's skin tone won't be dark enough for his or her tattoo. Smaller tattoos are easier to cover than large ones, and tattoos that have experienced raised scarring can be tricky to conceal fully. With some practice, using concealer and foundation can be an effective way to cover up tattoos on occasion.

Temporary Tattoos

Granted, a major allure of tattoos is their permanence. The fact that they can't be easily removed is the very reason why many people want to get them in the first place. However,

For thousands of years, henna has been used to create designs on the skin that are beautiful, natural, painless, and temporary.

for those who simply want to wear ink on their skin, a temporary tattoo is a great solution. Temporary tattoos can look amazing, and the best part is that they can be removed with little more than soap and water. It isn't a commitment. A person can get temporary tattoo after temporary tattoo in the same location.

At one time, these tattoos were little more than novelty items. Today, it's possible to get temporary tattoos that range from anywhere from $10 for several generic designs to thousands of dollars for custom work by a well-known artist. Most will last for a couple days unless efforts are taken to remove them. Temporary tattoos can also be a great way for people to test whether or not they really want a permanent tattoo. If they are comfortable with the attention they receive for having skin art, they might be good candidates for getting inked.

Henna

Henna has been used to dye hair and skin for thousands of years. In India, Pakistan, and Bangladesh, a paste made of the plant is applied to the arms and hands of brides, creating elaborate and beautiful designs. This art is known as mehndi. Women have mehndi done for weddings, festivals, and other special occasions. Henna is applied to the surface of the skin and is completely noninvasive.

After being applied to the skin, henna is allowed to set. Then the paste can be washed off. Although it isn't permanent, henna lasts for a while—usually for about two weeks. In its natural form, henna leaves a dark brown or dark orange mark on the skin. There are some forms of henna that come in different colors, but be warned that these are artificially colored. For instance, there is a demand for black henna, but there is no way to make it naturally. So companies add a number of synthetic chemicals in order to make this kind of henna, which some people can have allergic reactions to. For this reason, it's a good idea to test out any henna beforehand on a small patch of skin. After all, no one wants elaborate, henna-colored blisters on their arms and hands!

Regretting a Tattoo

In 2009, a Belgian eighteen-year-old named Kimberly Vlaminck went to a tattoo parlor to get inked…on her face. Her tattoo consisted of dozens of stars spreading over the left half of her face, going as far as the side of her nose. Her father flipped out when he saw the results, and she told him that she hadn't asked for so many stars. She said that she had actually fallen asleep during the tattoo process and woken up with a galaxy of fifty-six stars on her face. She attempted to sue the tattoo shop in order to get the money to have them removed. Vlaminck's claims were untrue, however. It turned out that she had indeed asked for the very tattoo she had gotten. The story broke internationally, making Kimberly Vlaminck one of the most infamous cases of tattoo regret. According to the *New York Daily News*, she had told reporters, "It is terrible for me. I cannot go out on to the street. I look like a freak."

When applying henna, it is important to make sure that the skin is clean, as dirt and natural skin oils can keep henna from having full contact with the skin. Body hair can also interfere with its application. Many people choose to have a professional apply henna, but it is possible to apply henna to one's own skin. Usually, a design is worked out and drawn on ahead of time. Some people use hectograph paper, which is a paper with dye on it, to transfer a design onto their skin. It's good to work out the design before applying the henna, since the skin starts absorbing it fairly quickly and mistakes will show up. Henna needs to set in order to properly stain the skin. This takes four to twelve hours. Some people use a hair dryer to speed up the process. Others put a sealant on their skin to help the henna set. The easiest method is to spray the design with hairspray.

Conclusion

Since tattoo removal is so painful, expensive, and time-consuming, what can be done to avoid it? There are two ways: The first is to not get any tattoos, and the second is to get a tattoo that won't cause regrets later on. Tattoo choices should be thought out very carefully. One simple way to prevent tattoo regret is to pick a design, get a copy of it, and hang it on the wall. If the design still seems appealing after six months, maybe it's OK to go ahead and start looking for a good tattoo artist to ink it. The design should still seem cool in a year, or even fifty years.

GLOSSARY

anesthetic A substance that provides relief from, or insensitivity to, pain.

carcinogenic Cancer-causing.

cataract A clouding of the eye's lens that often comes with age.

cauterize To seal skin by burning it.

dermabrasion The removal of skin with a spinning abrasive disc. Dermabrasion is meant to remove damaged skin so that new skin can grow back and replace it.

dermis The layer of skin protected by the epidermis, which holds the ink of a tattoo.

epidermis The outermost layer of skin.

excision A surgical procedure that involves cutting out the skin that holds a tattoo and closing up the wound.

henna A plant-based dye used to color skin and hair.

hygiene Practices promoting sanitary conditions.

incision In surgery, a cut made into the body.

India ink A simple black ink, made from black soot, that was traditionally used for drawing.

invasive Describing any kind of medical procedure that involves cutting into or inserting anything into the human body.

laser A generated beam of electromagnetic radiation.

mainstream Belonging to the culture shared by the majority of people.

pigment The matter in a cell or tissue that gives color in human skin.

procedure A specific medical operation.

scalpel A tool used by surgeons to make incisions.

scar A mark on the skin resulting from tissue regenerating after an injury. Scars stand out from the skin that surrounds them.

sterile Free of contaminates.

wound An injury that inflicts a cut or tear in the skin.

FOR MORE INFORMATION

Alliance of Professional Tattooists
215 West 18th Street, Suite 210
Kansas City, MO 64108
(816) 979-1300
Web site: http://www.safe-tattoos.com
The Alliance of Professional Tattooists is dedicated to providing information to artists and the public at large about tattooing.

Canadian Association of Professional Tattoo Artists
10359 82 Avenue NW
Edmonton, AB T6E 1Z9
Canada
(780) 413-7233
This association counts some of Canada's foremost tattoo artists among its members.

Centers for Disease Control and Prevention (CDC)
1600 Clifton Road
Atlanta, GA 30333
(800) 232-4636
Web site: http://www.cdc.gov
The CDC monitors public health issues and works to educate the public, enhance public safety, and promote healthy behavior. It is a source of information about any side effects resulting from tattoo removal.

Tattoo Archive
618 West 4th Street

Winston-Salem, NC 27101

(336) 722-4422

Web site: http://www.tattooarchive.com/contact_us.htm
The Tattoo Archive works to preserve tattoo history.

Tattoo Club of America

c/o Spider Webb's Studio

Captains Cove Seaport

1 Bastwick Avenue

Bridgeport, CT 06605

(203) 335-3992
This organization promotes the art of tattooing and maintains a library and tattoo museum.

Web Sites

Due to the changing nature of Internet links, Rosen Publishing has developed an online list of Web sites related to the subject of this book. This site is updated regularly. Please use this link to access the list:

http://www.rosenlinks.com/ttt/eti

For Further Reading

Barnes, Jennifer Lynn. *Tattoo*. New York, NY: Delacorte Press, 2007.

Currie-McGhee, L. K. *Tattoos and Body Piercing*. San Diego, CA: Lucent Publishing, 2005.

Cuyper, Christa de, and Maria Luisa Cotapos. *Dermatologic Complications with Body Art: Tattoos, Piercings and Permanent Make-Up*. New York, NY: Springer Publishing, 2010.

Finn, Ericka. *The Complete Guide to Tattoo Removal*. Pasadena, CA: Zibi Books, 2007.

Hudson, Karen L. *Living Canvas: Your Total Guide to Tattoos, Piercings, and Body Modification*. Berkeley, CA: Seal Press, 2009.

Kiesbye, Stefan. *Body Piercing and Tattoos*. New York, NY: Greenhaven Press, 2008.

Levin, Judith. *Tattoos and Indigenous Peoples*. New York, NY: Rosen Publishing, 2008.

Levy, Janey. *Tattoos in Modern Society*. New York, NY: Rosen Publishing, 2008.

Manning, Mick. *Under Your Skin: Your Amazing Body*. Park Ridge, IL: Albert Whitman & Company, 2007.

Nagle, Jeanne. *Tattoo Artists*. New York, NY: Rosen Publishing, 2008.

Pomaska, Anna. *Henna Hearts Tattoos*. Mineola, NY: Dover Publications, 2006.

Porterfield, Jason. *Tattoos and Secret Societies*. New York, NY: Rosen Publishing, 2008.

Reardon, John. *Getting a Tattoo: The Complete Idiot's Guide*. New York, NY: Penguin, 2008.

Rush, John A. *Spiritual Tattoo: A Cultural History of Tattooing, Piercing, Scarification, Branding, and Implants*. Berkeley, CA: Frog Books, 2005.

Sawyer, Sarah. *Body Piercing and Tattooing: The Hidden Dangers of Body Art*. New York, NY: Rosen Publishing, 2007.

Sawyer, Sarah. *Frequently Asked Questions About Body Piercing and Tattooing*. New York, NY: Rosen Publishing, 2008.

BIBLIOGRAPHY

Finn, Ericka. *The Complete Guide to Tattoo Removal.* Pasadena, CA: Zibi Books, 2007.

Grant, Tim. "Tattoos, Piercings Bad Sign for Job: Though Acceptance Is Growing, Many Firms Still Are Not Tolerant." *Detroit News*, August 19, 2010. Retrieved August 30, 2010 (http://detnews.com/article/20100819/BIZ/8190375/Tattoos--piercings-bad-sign-for-job#ixzz10NVBddYH).

Hudson, Karen L. *Living Canvas: Your Total Guide to Tattoos, Piercings, and Body Modification.* Berkeley, CA: Seal Press, 2009.

La Ferla, Ruth. "Tattooed for a Day, Wild for a Night." *New York Times*, January 24, 2008. Retrieved July 1, 2010 (http://www.nytimes.com/2008/01/24/fashion/24TATTOO.html).

Lineberry, Cate. "Tattoos: The Ancient and Mysterious History." Smithsonian.com, January 1, 2007. Retrieved July 1, 2010 (http://www.smithsonianmag.com/history-archaeology/tattoo.html).

Mayo Clinic. "Cosmetic Surgery: Dermabrasion at Mayo Clinic." 2010. Retrieved July 1, 2010 (http://www.mayoclinic.org/cosmetic-surgery/dermabrasion.html).

Nocera, Kate. "Teen Kimberly Vlaminck with 56 Star Tattoos on Her Face Admits She Wanted Them the Whole Time."

New York Daily News, June 23, 2009. Retrieved July 1, 2010 (http://www.nydailynews.com/news/national/2009/06/23/2009-06-23_teen_kimberly_vlaminck_with_56_star_tattoos_on_her_face_admits_she_wanted_them_t.html).

Padilla, Darcy. "Erasing Gang Tattoos from Faces and Hands." *New York Times*, May 8, 1994. Retrieved July 1, 2010 (http://www.nytimes.com/1994/05/08/us/erasing-gang-tattoos-from-faces-and-hands.html).

Reardon, John. *Getting a Tattoo: The Complete Idiot's Guide.* New York, NY: Penguin, 2008.

Singer, Natasha. "Erasing Tattoos, Out of Regret or for a New Canvas." *New York Times*, June 17, 2007. Retrieved July 1, 2010 (http://www.nytimes.com/2007/06/17/us/17tattoo.html?_r=1).

U.S. Food and Drug Administration. "Tattoos & Permanent Makeup." June 23, 2008. Retrieved July 1, 2010 (http://www.fda.gov/Cosmetics/ProductandIngredientSafety/ProductInformation/ucm108530.htm).

INDEX

About the Author

Frank Spalding is a writer from upstate New York. He has long been fascinated by the history of tattooing. When he was ten years old, he got his first temporary tattoo, the Egyptian god Set, which he applied to his forehead. He's very glad that it wasn't permanent.

Photo Credits